Essential Oils

Unleash the Power of Essential Oils Using this Proven Step by Step Guide

Table of Contents:

Introduction

I want to thank you and congratulate you for downloading the book, *"Essential Oils: Unleash the Power of Essential Oils Using this Proven Step by Step Guide"*.

This book contains proven steps and strategies on how to use essential oils for your various health and beauty issues, for your home, and for your pet's well-being.

Using essential oils is a great way to ensure that you are using all-natural ingredients for yourself and your home. They are cheaper compared to many commercial products but can be as effective. They are also very versatile. One bottle of just about any essential oil can be used in various ways as will be shown in this book.

Thanks again for downloading this book, I hope you enjoy it!

reparation, damages, or monetary loss due to the information herein, either directly or indirectly.

Respective authors own all copyrights not held by the publisher.

The information herein is offered for informational purposes solely, and is universal as so. The presentation of the information is without contract or any type of guarantee assurance.

The trademarks that are used are without any consent, and the publication of the trademark is without permission or backing by the trademark owner. All trademarks and brands within this book are for clarifying purposes only and are the owned by the owners themselves, not affiliated with this document.

Chapter 1 – Step 1 – Getting to Know Essential Oils

The first step in unleashing the power of essential oils is to know what they are, what they can do, and how to use them correctly.

What are essential oils?

Essential oils are, literally, the essential oils of plants. To explain, first, "essential" refers to the extracted essences of plants or certain plant parts. Chemically speaking, a plant is comprised of 3 substances: water, plant fiber or cellulose, and the plant's nutrients or essence. The essence is extracted from the plant either by boiling it and then distilling the resulting tea or by squeezing the plant then further distilling the squeezed juice. The plant's essence is what makes it that particular plant. Without it, all plants will be the same in chemical structure.

Second, "oil" refers to the fact that essential oils are hydrophobic substances which means they do not mix with water. A vigorous shake will make the essential oil combine with water, but eventually they will separate.

What can essential oils do or what are they used for? Essential oils can do whatever the plant can do. For example, sniffing the lavender plant can calm the nerves. Therefore, sniffing a drop of lavender essential oil can produce the same effect. After all, it is the essence of lavender which gives the calming effect. The only difference between the plant and its essential oil is the latter is concentrated.

How should essential oils be used?

It is first important to mention that essential oils are not simply artificially fragranced oils which some unscrupulous manufacturers like to label as "essential oil." Artificial fragrance oils are, as their name says, artificial, whereas essential oils are 100% natural. If you are using essential oils primarily for the plant nutrients rather than the fragrance, then using artificial fragrance oils will be futile. On the other hand, if you are using essential oils primarily for the fragrance, you can probably get away with using the high end artificial fragrance oils; but those with more discerning noses will claim that their scent is inferior. This will be discussed more in the succeeding chapters.

To know whether you are buying true essential oil or artificial fragrance oil, check the price. The former will be more expensive than the latter due to how it is manufactured. Recall that a plant is comprised of water, cellulose and its essence. About 95-99% of the plant is water and cellulose. This means you need a lot of plants to extract only a small amount of essential oil. For example, it takes about 11 pounds of lavender to make only 15 milliliters of essential oil. Given the amount of effort it takes to grow the lavender plant and the effort of extracting the oil, it would not make sense to pay only $1 for 15 milliliters of lavender essential oil (unless, of course, the store is having a major sale.)

A reasonable price for the more common essential oils like lavender is about $10 for 30 milliliters. The less common essential oils like frankincense will probably be more expensive because not a lot of manufacturers make them. The price will also depend on how difficult it is to extract the oil and/or how difficult it is to grow the plant. Further, essential oil that is extracted from organically grown plants will be double the price due to the complexities of organic farming.

To ensure that you are getting true essential oil, stick to the reputable brands and stores. They sell their oils in properly labeled bottles which state the scientific name of the plant, the country of origin or where the plant was grown, and the date of manufacture. They will also sell essential oils in dark, opaque bottles which prevent light from degrading the product. The label should state whether the essential oil has been diluted or not. The reasons why buying diluted essential oil may be a good idea will be discussed in the succeeding chapters.

The second point in using essential oils correctly is to know that *not* everything that is natural is harmless. People who make this mistake forget that many plants (e.g. poison ivy and poison oak) are harmful to humans, and some plants are deadly when ingested (e.g. yew tree). Several substances of animal origin are also deadly like the venom of some snake species.

Essential oils of poisonous plants are manufactured mainly for professional chemists, but sometimes, they can be bought by ordinary people from unscrupulous manufacturers. In this book, poisonous essential oils will not be mentioned. For the beginner, it is best to stick with essential oils which are proven safe like lavender, tea tree oil, and rose rather than to experiment with unknown varieties.

Further, a person can be allergic to a harmless natural substance, e.g. strawberries and nuts. Those who suffer from many allergies are usually told to avoid all essential oils, including the relatively safe ones like lavender. People with special medical conditions like pregnant and lactating women, those who are taking prescription medication, those who have asthma, etc. must also consult with their doctor before trying out essential oils.

The above advice is given not to scare you but just to help you be on the safe side. It is already know that certain substances, even if considered safe for most people, can interact with certain medications or affect a physical condition. For example, the over-the-counter acne medication salicylic acid is safe for non-pregnant and non-lactating women, but not safe otherwise.

For people who do not suffer from many allergies or do not have special medical conditions, essential oils are generally safe. However, it is still best to do an allergy test first. To do this, apply a tiny drop of essential oil on your skin, preferably in a "hidden" part of the body like behind the ear. If no irritation occurs after 24 hours, it means the essential oil is safe to use. If irritation occurs, the spot must be cleansed immediately and the essential oil must not be used.

Again, this advice is given not to scare or to deter you from using essential oils but to help ensure your safety. As mentioned, most people who do not suffer from allergies can use essential oils safely, but the human body can sometimes be unpredictable. A person might be the one out of a million who suffers from a unique allergy. If so, whatever benefit one may gain from the use of essential oil will be cancelled out.

The third point in using essential oils correctly is to know the proper way of using them depending on the purpose. They can be used in three ways: applied topically, inhaled as a scent, or ingested. These will be discussed in detail in the succeeding chapters.

Chapter 2 – Step 2 – Choosing the Right Essential Oil

The right essential oil to get will depend on three things: purpose, budget and personal preference.

Purpose

It was already stated in the introduction that essential oils can be used for various problems. Most people buy a bottle of essential oil only for one purpose, but it pays to know how many uses an essential oil can have.

To make things easier, this chapter will mention the purpose then list the essential oils which can be used for that.

Anti-bacterial for skin infections, wounds and acne for both humans and pets (topically applied): lavender, peppermint, eucalyptus, tea tree oil

Anti-bacterial essential oils can also be used for cleaning the home.

Calming/Decreases stress/Helps with insomnia (inhaled scent): lavender, chamomile, geranium, vetiver, tangerine, sandalwood, cedarwood, vanilla

Clears stuffy noses (inhaled scent): lavender, peppermint, eucalyptus

Clears dark spots on the skin (topically applied): lemon, chamomile, rose

Clears dandruff: tea tree oil, eucalyptus, peppermint

Decreases itch especially for eczema and psoriasis (topically applied): lavender, peppermint, eucalyptus, tea tree oil

Kills ticks, fleas and lice for both humans and pets (topically applied): lavender, peppermint, eucalyptus, tea tree oil

Increases concentration (inhaled scent): peppermint, jasmine

Increases energy (inhaled scent): lemon, grapefruit, and lime

Increases metabolism (when ingested): cinnamon, ginger, grapefruit, lemon, peppermint

Stimulates blood flow to the epidermis to aid in skin rejuvenation and hair growth (topically applied): lavender, peppermint, rose, geranium, sandalwood, rosemary, vanilla

Notice that several essential oils have more than one purpose. That is why it is possible to save money when using essential oils. There is no need to buy separate products for various needs. Also, since essential oils are, by definition, concentrated (unless they are labeled as diluted), only a small amount is used every time. A 30 milliliter bottle which costs $10 can last about a year depending on how it is used.

Notice too that lavender can be used for several purposes. That is why it is considered the universal essential oil. It is also considered the safest to use. Lavender allergy is very rare and most people with special medical conditions can use it. (However, as mentioned above, those with special medical conditions must check with the doctor first just to be on the safe side even if they will only use lavender.)

Budget

As mentioned previously, essential oils may vary in price for various reasons. It is up to the consumer to decide whether paying extra money is worth it. Take note that the more expensive essential oil is not, generally speaking, necessarily more effective. For example, both lavender and rose essential oils are effective for skin rejuvenation, but rose is more expensive because more plants are needed to make the same amount of essential oil. However, since every human body is unique, perhaps one's experience may prove that rose is more effective than lavender for this particular purpose making the increased price worth it.

Personal Preference

Of course, people will always choose what they enjoy using. If your experience has shown that both lavender and rose are effective but you simply prefer the scent of rose, then it makes sense for you to buy rose essential oil instead.

Chapter 3 – Step 3 – Combining Essential Oils

There are two reasons why essential oils are combined: to obtain more benefits and to create a more pleasant scent.

To obtain more benefits

It is sometimes more convenient to combine two or more essential oils which are used for different purposes to avoid the need to apply different products separately. For example, if someone wishes to remove dark spots from the skin for a more even complexion *and* to stimulate blood flow to help retain a youthful glow, she can choose to use rose essential oil which is effective for both purposes. However, if this person dislikes the scent of rose, she can use a combination of lemon and lavender. Instead of applying the two essential oils separately, it is more convenient to combine the two in equal amounts then store the solution in a separate container.

To create a more pleasant scent

You might grow bored of having only one essential oil and its particular scent; thus, it is a good idea to create a different scent.

Combining essential oils to create a different scent is not easy. Professional perfumers must study for several years before they get their recipes right, but beginners can try these simple scent combinations:

- 1:1 lavender and lemon
- 1:1 rose and sandalwood
- 2:2:1 rose, sandalwood and vanilla
- 1:1 vanilla and jasmine
- 2:2:1 rosemary, peppermint and grapefruit

Take note, though, that when using essential oils for aromatherapy, i.e. obtaining the benefits of essential oils through inhaling their scent, combined essential oils will provide combined benefits. For example, vanilla is calming while jasmine increases concentration. This may be a good combination for students who are stressed and find it difficult to study, but it is not a good combination for insomnia sufferers since the jasmine might keep them awake.

More information about essential oil fragrance recipes can be found from books and websites about perfumes.

Still on the subject of aromatherapy, it was mentioned in chapter 1 that high end artificial fragrance oils can sometimes be used instead of essential oils. These are less expensive than true essential oils and smell almost like the real thing, but discerning noses, especially those who are used to the scent of true essential oils, might be able to notice a slight difference.

Under no circumstances should cheap artificial fragrance oils be used. These are sold very cheaply, perhaps less than $1 for a small bottle, and can be found in the home décor section of most discount stores. These fragrances are more likely to cause headaches than provide anything beneficial.

Chapter 4 – Step 4 – To Dilute or not to Dilute

As mentioned in chapter 1, essential oils can be sold either pure, i.e. 100% strength, or diluted. Essential oils can be diluted with clean water, preferably distilled, alcohol, aloe vera gel, plant oils like olive or argan, or other ingredients. Diluted products must be labeled as such and the strength or percentage of the essential oil must be indicated in the label.

Essential oils can also be an ingredient in commercial shampoos, bath soaps, laundry detergents and household cleansers. Likewise, essential oils can be found in make-up and skin moisturizers. Obviously, the essential oil here will be diluted, but since these products are marketed mainly as cleansers and skin products rather than as essential oils, the percentage of oil used is usually not mentioned.

The reason essential oil is sometimes sold diluted depends on what it is marketed as. For example, a product that is labeled as "tea tree oil antibacterial spray" which is marketed for use on the hands will obviously be diluted tea tree oil. Using pure tea tree oil on the hands will result in an overwhelming scent which some people may find irritating. Since tea tree oil is still effective against bacteria at 5% concentration, the product is not falsely labeled, but it cannot be used for other purposes like killing ticks and fleas. 5% tea tree oil is no longer effective for that purpose.

A product with 5% tea tree oil will be cheaper than a bottle of 100% tea tree oil. It is also convenient for some consumers who can't be bothered to make their own tea tree oil spray. Whether or not to buy diluted essential oil products for whatever reason remains a personal preference. However, take note that in the long run, buying pure essential oil and diluting it according to how it will be used will save more money if the same bottle of essential oil is used for various purposes, e.g. to make antibacterial spray, to be applied topically on acne, to kill the dog's fleas, etc.

For those who choose to buy bottles of pure essential oils, they must know when to dilute it and when not to, and how.

The general rules for knowing whether or not to dilute essential oils are as follows:

For topical application: Dilute or keep pure according to skin, nose, and eye sensitivity.

Some individuals can tolerate the scent of pure essential oils, but some can't. The exceptions are pets and children. Since their skin is more sensitive than adult humans' skin, essential oils must always be diluted.

What about the correct percentage? How strong must the diluted solution be? Here, only trial and error can tell. The solution must be weak enough to prevent irritation but strong enough to still be effective. The correct percentage will vary depending on the individual.

For use in oil burners or room sprays: Always dilute.

Essential oils must never be heated undiluted in oil burners because direct heat will alter its scent. They must also never be sprayed directly into the atmosphere like in the case of room sprays because the scent will be too strong. Dark colored essential oils may also stain when sprayed undiluted on fabric.

For ingestion to increase metabolism: always dilute. Consuming pure essential oil can irritate the surfaces of the tongue and the mouth. The taste of pure essential oil may also be unpleasant.

Meanwhile, the general rule for *how* to dilute essential oil is this: Dilute according to how it will be applied or used.

To be used as a skin or room spray: Dilute with clean water or 50% ethyl or isopropyl alcohol. If the spray will be used topically, take note that alcohol can dry the skin. Start with 5 drops per cup of liquid and adjust according to the desired scent or effectivity. Shake well before every use.

To be used on the skin: Dilute with liquid plant oils, e.g. jojoba, argan, olive, etc. will result in a liquid formula; solid plant oils, e.g. virgin coconut oil, or seed butters, e.g. cocoa butter, will result in a cream formula. Natural waxes like beeswax can also be used. Essential oils can be mixed with liquid oils directly, but solid oils, butters and waxes must be melted over a low heat first to allow the even distribution of the essential oil.

Take note that some plant oils and waxes can alter the scent of the essential oil. To avoid this, use a neutral smelling oil like grape seed oil or a neutral smelling wax like unscented soy wax. If using artificial wax is not an issue, unscented petroleum jelly is a cheap option.

However, it is possible to combine certain oils and waxes to create a pleasant scent combination. For example, if vanilla essential oil is used for skin rejuvenation, diluting it with cocoa butter will result in a chocolate scented cream. Another good combination is lemon and beeswax for a honey lemon scent.

For those with oilier skins or for those who dislike the emollient feel of oils, butters, and waxes, aloe vera gel can be used for dilution. Water, concentrated black or green tea (steep 1 tea bag in ¼ cup boiling water and allow to cool), and ethyl or isopropyl alcohol are also good choices for oily skins. This will result in a toner-like product which must be applied with a cotton ball or sprayed on the skin.

Start with 5 drops of essential oil per cup of liquid oil, seed butter, or wax and adjust according to need and preference.

Alternatively, as was explained earlier, essential oils can also be used pure if the individual is not sensitive.

Essential oils can also be mixed with shampoo and liquid soap to gain the benefits while cleansing the skin. For example, since rosemary essential is good for stimulating hair growth, it may be added to shampoo. Use 10 drops per 1 liter of shampoo or liquid soap and adjust according to sensitivity and effectivity.

To be used as a topical rinse or soak: Dilute with clean water. Use 15 drops per gallon of water and adjust according to sensitivity and effectivity.

To be used as a disinfecting solution for household surfaces: 20 drops of any antibacterial essential oil per gallon of water is enough to disinfect non-porous surfaces.

To disinfect the laundry: Add 20 drops of any antibacterial essential oil to the water used to rinse a small load of laundry.

Alternatively, 10 drops of antibacterial essential oil can be added to each cup of powdered or liquid detergent.

IMPORTANT: Do not apply the essential oil directly on the clothes since it may stain.

To scent potpourri: Add 5 drops to 1 cup of potpourri and mix well to distribute the essential oil evenly.

An alternative to potpourri is baking soda. The essential oil will scent the room while the baking soda will absorb bad odors.

For use in oil burners: Use 1 drop of essential oil for every tablespoon of water in the burner's bowl.

For scenting candles: At least 20 drops of essential oil must be used per pound of candle wax. Anything less will result in a scent that is too subtle to detect.

For bar soap making: For each 100 gram bar of soap, add 10 drops of essential oil.

To be ingested: Add the essential oil to any liquid that can be safely ingested. The essential oil can also be combined with other ingredients while cooking. For example, cinnamon essential oil can be used instead of powdered cinnamon.

IMPORTANT: The maximum amount of essential oil each person can intake for this purpose is 2 drops a day. Start with 1 drop a day then move up to 2 drops a day if no discomfort occurs. Go back to 1 drop a day if 2 drops cause discomfort. Also, stick to the recommended essential oils. Other essential oils besides those mentioned in chapter 2 for this purpose might be harmful if ingested.

Also, using essential oils this way will only slightly increase one's metabolism to aid in weight loss, though this method will not be enough to offset an unhealthy diet and lifestyle.

Lastly, it is important that only essential oils are ingested and not artificial fragrance oils. It will be better to buy essential oils for ingestion from cooking supply stores to be sure that the product is 100% safe to be eaten by humans.

Conclusion

Thank you again for downloading this book!

I hope this book was able to help you to know how to unleash the power of essential oils for various purposes.

The next step is to try out the tips listed here to know which works for you. Remember to always be mindful of the precautions mentioned in this book.

Finally, if you enjoyed this book, then I'd like to ask you for a favor, would you be kind enough to leave a review for this book on Amazon? It'd be greatly appreciated!

Thank you and good luck!

www.ingramcontent.com/pod-product-compliance
Lightning Source LLC
Chambersburg PA
CBHW061953280526
45787CB00004B/1843